Essential Oils: Your Beginners Guide to Essential Oils and Aromatherapy

Sally Evans

Contents

Introduction

If you're looking to get started with essential oils you want to make sure that you're doing it right. Of course, if you've never used essential oils before then you're going to want to make sure that you know what they really are and how they should be used.

In this book we're going to talk about all of that and more. We're going to help you understand what essential oils are, what aromatherapy is, how it works and what products you can and should use for it. We'll even talk about how to use different oils for different needs.

If you're looking for a way to get yourself feeling better, looking better and being more productive then you're definitely going to want to check this out. Make sure that you look at the essential oils that are going to help most with your needs and then make sure that you are really using them in your life.

You'll be surprised what you can accomplish with just a few simple oils. They're going to really change your life and all that with just something that's also going to smell great in your home and on you as well. So let's get started with what these oils are and what they can do for you.

Chapter 1: What is an Essential Oil?

The Basics

Essential oils are the extracted oils of a plant. They can come from any plant at all and typically carry on the fragrance of that plant as well as a variety of healing benefits associated with the plant itself.

The plant needs to be distilled in order to produce this oil and each plant that is used actually only produces a very tiny amount. It actually takes literal tons of each plant to make as little as one pound of essential oil.

That's the main reason that each little bottle that you buy is going to be so expensive. Because it takes so much to make you are actually getting charged for all of the plants that have to be sacrificed for the process. You're also paying for all the hard work that goes into the process.

Originally, essential oils were believed to be the spirit of a plant. These spirits were believed to have mystical healing powers that could cure a variety of different ailments. Though we've come to understand now that there really isn't anything 'spiritual' about essential oils, we do know that our ancestors were right in believing that these oils had healing powers.

They really can provide you with a lot of different benefits and healing abilities in a range of different parts of the body and in plenty of different ways. They can provide help with weight loss, health and anything else you can think of through several different methods we'll explain later.

While in the plant these oils actually serve an important purpose:

They help to attract bees and other insects which help to pollinate the plant, making it grow even better. This is believed to occur because of the aroma of the oil.

They also help to prevent other plants from growing too close, thereby stealing the nutrients from the first plant. This occurs because of the chemicals that are a natural part of these oils and prevent other plant species from popping up.

Next, they can help to keep other animals and insects from eating the plant because of the chemicals and also because of the smell itself. These can be dangerous (or just taste bad) to plant predators.

Finally, they are antifungal and antibacterial and therefore can keep many diseases out of the plant beds and therefore keep the plant healthy and living longer.

Shopping for Essential Oils Step by Step

When you're looking to purchase an essential oil you want to make sure that it really is what it says it is. This means you need to look at a variety of different features of the product in order to be sure that it will provide what you need, therapeutic benefits.

1. Look at the Price. Does it seem inexpensive compared to other websites or stores you've looked at? Pure essential oils are not cheap so you want to be suspicious of anything that says it's a pure oil but seems a lot cheaper than anything else you've seen.

2. Look at the Label. Does it actually say "Pure _____ Oil?" If it does then you can move on with the other steps, if it doesn't you'll want to walk away.

   Pure extract is going to be more expensive but it's much better for your purposes if you dilute it yourself rather than purchasing anything that's already been diluted.

   Also look to see if the label states it is therapeutic grade. You don't want anything less because that's how you're going to get the benefits you want.

3. Look at the Bottle. What is the bottle made of? If it's made out of glass then you're possibly safe. If it's made of plastic you want to keep looking. Plastic is not sufficient to keep essential oils in. It has to be stored in glass to be stored properly so make sure the product you're looking at has that distinction.

4. Look at the Name. It should specifically say therapeutic oil or at least *not* say anything like fragrance or aroma. These are clues that what you're actually buying is a type of perfume or fragrance rather than being the therapeutic tool that you're actually looking for.

   Be sure it also has a true botanical name. You may have to do a little research to find out the specific name. You can look for it somewhere on the bottle as well. The botanical name will only be included if it's authentic.

Word of Caution

Make sure you're getting real essential oils when you go shopping since there are plenty of fakes out there. You're definitely going to have to spend a lot to get the quality products but if you don't get pure essential oil that really is what you're looking for you're not going to get the therapeutic benefits that you're looking for.

A true essential oil is going to cost you some money and it's going to fit all the information we talked about above. If it doesn't you should keep looking.

Essential oils could cost you a large amount of money if you aren't careful. Make sure that you're paying attention to the price per ounce. You don't want to get up to the counter or check out online and realize that you've just spent thousands of dollars on one bottle of essential oils (and that's entirely possible to do).
You don't need a lot of oil in order to carry out any of our processes that we're going to discuss so make sure you are buying only what

you really need and not purchasing large quantities that are going to cost you a small fortune. You'll be able to get plenty of use out of a small bottle so don't get discouraged.

Exercise #1

Take a trip to an herbalist store near you. There is probably one close by that sells alternative therapies and health products. You may even have an aromatherapy store or a massage parlor that sells their own oils.

Take a few minutes to look around at everything they have and familiarize yourself with what they look like and even what they smell like. Talking to the owner of the store (or skipping ahead to the last chapter in this book) will give you a better idea of which oils are best for which ailments or needs.

Try to figure out which ones might be best for your needs or for stress relief. We'll help you out more in later chapters but for now see if you can figure it out.

Chapter 2: What is Aromatherapy?

The Basics

Aromatherapy is using plant extracts and oils to help someone feel better or actually be better as far as their health goes. It is often used by people who suffer from health conditions such as being overweight or by people who are looking for a new way to relax when they find themselves in a stressful environment.

The different types of aromas can be used in a number of different ways (and of course there are a lot of them around).

If you're looking to get into aromatherapy you want to consider all those different scents that are available. We all know that the number of different types of plants in the world is unknown but believed to be extremely large.

What this means is you have a huge pool of plants that you can choose from to help you feel healthier and happier in your life. Choosing the right one isn't always easy but we'll help you understand some of the best ones for a few more common conditions as we go along.

The Use of Essential Oils Evolution

Now, in order to use aromatherapy the right way you need to understand what it really is about. It originated in 1937, at least the word did. No one knows when humans first started using some type of aromatherapy to help themselves in these ways.

What we do know is Rene Gattefosse created the term aromatherapy and started working with oils as a way of healing different ailments in his clients. A perfumer and chemist by trade, Rene had no medical training but he was able to create a way to help others feel better in ways they hadn't expected.

So what does the term aromatherapy actually mean? Well, from reading the book that Rene created and following what he did with his clients and patients we assume that the meaning he created was for application of essential oils for a type of holistic healing in a therapeutic way.

Of course, it's impossible to ask him now, but this seems to have been his intention from the way that he encouraged others to use the essential oils. Of course, now we see aromatherapy as a way of treating not just the mind and spirit but the entire body as well.

Word of Caution

Now, it's important to note that not all essential oils are intended to work for everyone. It's also important to note that not all plants are going to produce positive essential oils. There are a number of plants out there in the world that are poisonous and even deadly if you touch or ingest them (not that you're supposed to ingest your essential oils anyway).
Make sure that you are not picking just any plant and trying to create your own essential oils. You want to purchase them from a reputable place and make sure that you know what you're getting at all times.

Exercise #2

For this chapter take some time to do a little research. Look online and see what you can find about different essential oils. Look at the number of different types of oils there actually are. You may be surprised how many different types are available.

Try to find a website or a book that lists every essential oil we know as of right now (as a hint there's a glossary in the back of this book). Just look at how many essential oils there are and then look at the number of plants believed to be in existence in the world. You'll definitely see what we mean when we say that essential oils are all around us.

Chapter 3: How to Use Essential Oils

What You'll Learn

Now, using essential oils properly is extremely important to being able to feel the benefits of them. You need to understand what these oils are meant for and how they are going to work best.

So in this chapter we're going to help you understand a little more about how to use essential oils so that when you get to your next chapters, the ones that are going to talk to you about the right essential oils for you, you're going to know what to do with them to get the best benefits.

There are several different ways that you can actually use essential oils. By definition these are liquid forms of the essence of a plant and so, they can be used in many different application methods as well as simply being placed in a specific area.

You've probably tried candles, plug-ins and other forms of scented products in your home before (even food) and you've noticed that you like certain ones better than others or that you feel more relaxed with some than others. This is similar to what you will get with essential oils.

The Different Uses of Essential Oils

1. One of the common methods for using essential oils is to massage with them. If you go to a massage parlor or even if you are at home with a friend or partner you can use essential oils in place of traditional massage oil.

    In fact, even traditional massage oils will usually have at least a little of the essential oils in them because they help you to relax. The process of massage is not their only tool to relieve stress, the scent of the oils that they use work too.

2. Personal care products are another way to use essential oils. You can actually create your own shampoo, body wash, bath salts, lotions or even compresses that are infused with essential oils. This helps aid in the inhalation of those oils and it will improve the way that you feel and also what you are able to experience.

   You're going to feel far more relaxed this way and you won't even have to change your routine. All you do is follow your normal daily process and you start feeling better right away. You'll also be able to breathe this throughout the day with many of these methods which can help.

3. Next, you can inhale the essential oils through diffusers, evaporation, steam or spray. Remember to keep your concentration low (we'll discuss this more later) and you'll actually be surprised what you feel.

   You will get a reasonable amount of the oil on you or near you and this will help you to breathe it in. This is great for your home, even if you're not there, because you'll be able to smell the oils when you arrive at home. This means you get instant relief from your stress during the day when you walk in your door.

4. Finally, these oils can actually be used for wound care. If you have a cut, a bruise, a bite or anything else you can actually use the oils to help treat those wounds. Keep in mind the types of oils that you're using because not all of them are going to be good for wounds.

   Some may even hurt your healing process or hurt you when applied. Open wounds especially should be treated with care and you need to be careful of the amount and type of essential oils that you use on them.

Example

If you're going to use essential oils for massage you want to create a blend with traditional massage oil. For adults you want to use one drop of the oil compared to one teaspoon of the actual oil. If you're using these types of oils with your children you want even less.

For children who are older than 2 you can use the same concentration but infants should have 1 drop to 4 teaspoons of regular oil and toddlers should have 1 drop per 2 teaspoons of regular oil. You would then rub the oil gently into the skin.

Word of Caution

Now we said you don't want to ingest your essential oils but this isn't always the case. What you want to do is talk with a doctor before you ingest any of these oils. They can be beneficial for your health but only if your doctor says that it is safe and healthy.

Some may interact with medical conditions or medications and you want to make sure that you are aware of the effects before you attempt this method. Make sure your doctor knows what you are taking and how much.

Exercise #3

For this exercise try a massage. You don't need to get an essential oil for this. Instead, just light a candle, burn some incense or put in some type of air freshener so you get a little of the scent during the process. You'll feel the benefits of what scent, mixed with the massage process really can do for you and you'll definitely be glad that you tried it.

The massage is going to relax your muscles but the scent is going to help relax your mind. If you don't relax both you're not going to feel completely stress free and you won't be able to get the health benefits that aromatherapy is going to offer.

Chapter 4: Using Essential Oils for Weight Loss

What You'll Learn

Here we're going to talk about some of the best essential oils if you're attempting to lose weight. Of course, the oils themselves are not going to do all of the work, but they are definitely going to aid in your work.

You won't feel as stressed about the process but you're also not going to feel as hungry either and some will even help you with your weight loss. There are a lot of things that essential oils can do for your weight loss ability. You may actually be surprised about all the things that you find.

The Best Essential Oils for Weight Loss

There are several essential oils that you can use for weight loss and they each have different abilities when it comes to helping you lose weight. You want to make sure that you're checking out different ones.

Of course, it's not difficult to take essential oils but you really want to make sure that you choose the right one based on your needs and your body. Remember that you should keep your doctor in the loop, especially if you're ingesting any of these oils, so you know if any will interact with your health conditions or medications.

Grapefruit Oil

This oil is actually great for your weight loss because it reduces oxidative damage in your body (which helps you lose weight) and also helps you to lower your cholesterol. The reason for this is that it helps your body break down fatty acids for energy.

That means you'll also feel more energized so you can get more exercise. You'll also get additional benefits from this oil including improved metabolism, Vitamin C, antioxidants, and the removal of toxins from your body. So you can improve your health immensely with this oil.

Peppermint Oil

Now this is a great oil because it helps you get rid of your appetite and your cravings as well. Now that doesn't mean you're not going to eat. What this means is you're going to feel like you don't need as much food. When you don't eat as much, you're not going to gain as much weight.

It's actually been proven that you can get these benefits just from inhaling the peppermint oil, without needing to ingest it. If you do ingest it however, you'll have other benefits such as digestive problems and you'll get a lot of omega-3 fatty acids, potassium, iron and magnesium (all good for your body).

Lemon Oil

This oil is similar to the grapefruit oil. It helps to get rid of intestinal parasites and also helps you improve your metabolism. You'll even get a lot of energy (which are two traits you get from grapefruit oil as well).

Another benefit is that you won't hold onto toxins or fat cells in your body. By massaging this oil into areas of cellulite you can get these benefits, though you can also get them through ingesting the oil in water.

Bergamot Oil

This is a type of Italian citrus fruit and it's great if you start feeling a little bit stressed about your weight loss (or weight gain). You want to make sure that if you're upset you use this oil for reducing your stress eating.

It will even help you reduce blood fat production, increase your metabolism and reduce the amount of cholesterol that's absorbed into your body. You can use this by inhaling it or even by eating it.

If you use it as a massage oil on your feet or neck you'll also be able to reduce the level of stress you feel.

Cinnamon Bark Oil

If you take in cinnamon bark you're actually going to feel full faster when you eat. You won't gain weight because you're going to eat less. Now this doesn't necessarily help you lose weight but you're going to be able to keep your weight more stable.

You won't build up as much sugar or fatty acids and you'll be able to improve your immune system and blood circulation (which can help to make you healthier than ever). You even get anti-inflammatory benefits.

Sandalwood Oil

This is very similar oil to bergamot oil. It helps you reduce the amount of eating that you do so you don't eat just because you're stressed. You also don't have to worry about negative feelings and emotions because of the oil as well.

You can take in this oil by inhaling it or by applying it to your stomach or feet. You can even add some of it to some honey or coconut milk to ingest it. Take it up for yourself and make sure you pick your favorite way that you can use it.

Example

There are plenty of different oils that you can use for your weight loss goals. So the important thing is to make sure that you are choosing the exact one that you want. Make sure that you are considering all of the benefits and make sure you think about what you really need. It's also important to consider the different scents.

If you don't like the scent or the taste you won't want to use that oil because it's not going to do you a lot of good. Think about it, if you absolutely hate the taste of onions and someone told you to eat onions would they make you feel calmer? Probably not. You still wouldn't like them. So you want to choose oils that you like.

Word of Caution

You should know that using the exact same oil over and over again is not going to help you as much as you might think. You want to make sure you alternate between different oils so you will get the actual benefits you want rather than taking the same thing over and over.

First you'll get bored after a while and second you're going to miss out on some things. Your oils aren't going to do as much if they simply stockpile in your body. They need time to work their way through. By alternating through a couple different oils you'll get better benefits a lot faster.

Exercise #4

For this exercise try out a variety of different oils. Think about what you need for your weight loss the most. Are you more interested in losing weight or are you looking for a way to reduce your stress eating?

You want to make sure you find one that you enjoy smelling or ingesting as well. Consider everything about these oils and determine one or two that you really like. That's how you're going to get the best benefits, if you enjoy the oil you're using.

Chapter 5: Using Essential Oils for Stress & Anxiety

What You'll Learn

One of the other big things that hurt a lot of people is stress & anxiety. Everyone feels these at some point in time or another but sometimes you may experience even more stress or anxiety than you can deal with.

You want to make sure that you are doing something about this. You have probably heard before that scents can make you feel better and you've probably experienced it as well. So just take some time to find a scent you really enjoy.

Oils for Stress & Anxiety

Lavender Oil

This oil is actually really good for a lot of different things. You'll get a calming, relaxing feeling and you'll also have a great pain reliever and antiseptic. You can use it if you have muscle pain or if you have any kind of injury from burns and cuts to bug bites.

The scent is great because it's light, floral, fresh and earthy all at the same time. You'll be able to feel better just because you get a good scent and then you'll get the added benefit from the health properties of the oil.

Frankincense Oil

A little more exotic, frankincense is great for stress relief because of the warm aroma that it gives off. It can even help with respiratory problems. That means you'll experience relief from asthma, coughing or even bronchitis.

So if you have any of these conditions or even if you have minor health problems like scars you can apply this oil and you'll actually be able to heal much faster. This is a great oil for those who love a little bit of variance in their oil scents.

Rose Oil

This oil is actually quite expensive but it's also one of the best you're likely to find. With the ability to reduce symptoms of eczema and menopause, this oil can also reduce stress and depression so you feel better about yourself.

You'll also be able to feel less stressed because of this oil and you can use it in any way you want. Just understand that you're going to pay a little more for this oil simply because it takes a whole lot of roses to make a very tiny amount of the oil. Even still it can definitely be worth it.

Chamomile Oil

The Roman version of this oil is the best one for mental anxiety and paranoia so it's actually going to help you improve your stress levels as well as your feelings about yourself. On the other hand, the German version of this particular oil is going to help you with any type of skin problems.

You can use it topically for this use and can inhale or ingest it for other uses. The best thing is you're going to get calming benefits and digestive assistance from either one of these no matter how you decide to take it in.

Vanilla Oil

The last oil we're going to talk about for stress and anxiety relief is vanilla. Now you've probably had the opportunity to smell vanilla quite frequently. It's actually a great oil for just about anything. It's popular for candles as well as car fresheners and home oils.

The essential oils will help with mental clarity as well as relieving upset stomach and increasing your relaxation. You'll even feel less cravings because you get the benefits of a sweet treat from the scent without actually taking in any sweets. As a result, you eat less junk food and feel better about yourself and your weight.

Example

These oils can be used in any way you want. You have the ability to take them in mixed with water, tea or honey or you can massage them into your skin to help you relax. One of the easiest things you can do is simply put them into a diffuser and allow yourself to relax while you breathe them in.

Even if you don't have the time or ability to actually stop what you're doing to take in the oils you can use them while you are working because you'll still be able to feel better about your abilities and relaxation.

Word of Caution

These oils are very potent and that means you're going to reduce the strength of them with a carrier oil when you're using them for ingestion or for anything else.

If you're applying them to your skin you also need to make sure that you're lowering the content and the strength because it can be dangerous if you're not careful and you use something too potent. You may find yourself feeling ill, especially if you use non-organic oils, which can contain chemicals.

Exercise #5

For this chapter you want to go out and try some different oils. You don't have to actually purchase an oil at this point but you should take the opportunity to try out different ones. Go to a candle store or an oil store and smell the different oils.

They're all going to give you similar benefits as far as stress relief but you want to make sure that you get something that has other benefits you can use as well. This is going to help you feel better overall. Try to find one or a couple that you really like the scent of and then weigh out the other benefits.

Chapter 6: Using Essential Oils for Mind Clarity

What You'll Learn

Have you found yourself forgetting things frequently? If you have then you know how frustrating it can be. Well there are actually essential oils that you can use to help improve your ability to remember things.

The important thing is to make sure that you use those oils properly and that you are getting the best ones. Improving your mind clarity is going to improve your ability to live your life the way that you want to. So make sure you take some time to get your mind going the way it should be.

Step by Step Description

Rosemary Oil

This oil is actually very popular because it has many benefits. It will help you feel healthier and it also works great if you add it to foods as well as using it for massage or diffusers. You'll be able to improve your overall health with it and you're also going to feel a lot sharper in your mind as well because it helps to activate different parts of your brain that improve your memory.

You don't want to spend your life struggling to remember important things after all, so take the time to develop better memory and definitely to make sure that your overall well-being is going to be improved however you can.

Basil Oil

This oil is great for helping to refresh your mind. You'll feel better in general and you'll find plenty of ways that you can use this oil for yourself. You'll be able to use it as a spice in many different food dishes and you can use it in more traditional methods as massage oil as well.

The great thing about this oil is that it's much more familiar, which means you will not have to get used to a completely different scent in your home. It's something that most people have smelled before and do not have a problem with (also important if you have someone with allergies in your home).

Bergamot Oil

This oil is great for your mind because it will help you to relax your mind. This is why it's also great for stress relief. But one thing many people don't realize is that stress can cause you to forget things as well.

If you are careful to reduce your stress levels by using this oil you'll also be able to help improve your memory at the same time. You will feel calmer as you go through your daily life and you're definitely going to feel a lot better about the way you accomplish things in your life. This oil can also be used in any way that you want from massage to diffuser.

Peppermint Oil

With its benefits to your digestion and intestines as well as the benefits it offers to your mind clarity, this oil is actually an all-around favorite. It has a lot to offer and it can definitely improve the way that you think and remember different things.

You want to consider the great benefits of this oil in regards to all aspects of health as well as to mental clarity. It's far more than just a one-trick pony after all, it helps with nearly any health condition that you might have when applied or ingested.

Cardamom Oil

Capable of improving your mind as well as relieving mental tiredness, this oil is also great for reducing nervousness as well as improving your ability to break down foods. It helps to protect the stomach when you eat anything so that you don't suffer from damage or from stomach conditions.

You'll feel better just from inhaling this oil though it's also great to use through ingestion as well. In fact, spices are made from this same plant which can help to improve the stomach conditions and digestion as well. It's just one of the many oils that will help your entire body.

Example

If you want to improve your mind then the best thing you can do is use these oils as a tool. Work through the project or work you need while you're burning the oils or using them in some type of diffuser.

You'll find that you feel smarter almost instantly and you'll definitely get those proverbial juices flowing at the same time. The key is to make sure that you are really taking in those oils and improving your mind all at the same time because you want to get the benefits as quickly as possible. A diffuser is going to be your best method.

Word of Caution

You're not going to instantly become smarter than you were before you used the oils. What you need to do is make sure that you use them somewhat regularly. Of course, you don't want to use them daily because they won't actually be as effective this way.

What you want to do instead is come up with a regular schedule of when you're going to use them and when you won't. This way you're going to improve your overall mind without also burning yourself out on the oils that are going to help you the most.

Exercise #6

Take some time to try out different scents to see which ones really speak to you. Some oils are going to make you feel more energized and ready to take on anything while others are going to make you feel a little bit more relaxed.

If you're looking to improve your overall mind clarity and your ability to not only remember but accomplish tasks then you are definitely going to want to get oil (or a couple oils) that make you feel more energized and awake. That's the only way you're going to improve your mind.

For this exercise actually use the oils. Instead of using a substitute for the oil you want to actually purchase a small vial of oil that you believe will really work for you.

Maybe you want to go to a store that sells these oils and smell them first or go to a candle store and get an idea of the scent before you order one. What you really want to do however is take it home and use it when you're working.

If you can use it at your job that's great but even using it just at home before you work on something is going to help you improve your focus. Make sure you use the right quantities for your needs and try using it in a diffuser near you when you're working.

Chapter 7: Using Essential Oils for Beauty

What You'll Learn

Everyone wants to make themselves look as good as they possibly can. You want to be your absolute best and that means making yourself beautiful. So how do you go about making yourself look more beautiful? Well it's actually not as difficult as you may think.

What you need to do is use some of the best essential oils in a topical manner to help improve your skin and improve your body overall. These oils can frequently be ingested as well which can improve your body from the inside out (which makes you look and feel better).

Step by Step Description

Frankincense Oil

Anti-bacterial in nature, this oil is also anti-inflammatory, meaning it's great for any kind of injury to the skin. Even if you have acne this can be a great oil to use because it helps to reduce the visibility of pores as well as helping to balance out your skin tone.

If you have wrinkles, scars or dry skin this will also help to improve your cell growth and get rid of dead skin cells, as well as helping keep your current skin cells much healthier than before. You're going to look a lot better just by using this oil topically to improve your skin.

Geranium Oil

Capable of balancing out the oils that are produced naturally by your body, this oil also helps you get rid of acne by making your skin healthier. For those with wrinkles this oil will make skin more elastic, causing fewer wrinkles to develop and will also help to tighten up your skin which makes existing wrinkles fade away.

If you have trouble with circulation or with any type of skin disease or wounds you're able to apply this oil directly over the area and you'll see benefits almost immediately. It's really great for just about anything that ails you.

Lavender Oil

With its great scent, lavender oil is also perfect for rejuvenating the skin. You'll have much better skin cells which will result in less wrinkles, less sun spots and a lot less scaring.

You won't have to worry about most of the signs of getting older because you're going to have all of these benefits that include relaxation and a better ability to relate to stressful situations. You'll feel a lot better and you're going to look a lot better because of all the changes to your skin that are going to happen with these essential oils.

Myrrh Oil

Exotic and old oil, myrrh has benefits for those who are starting to age. It will change the skin tone, improve the firmness of your skin and even help reduce the appearance of lines and wrinkles.

You won't have to worry as much about sun damage or about things like dry skin or rashes. If you have any type of medical problems, such as burns, cuts or bruises this oil also has some great anti-inflammatory properties. These are going to improve the look and feel of your skin. You'll be surprised just how quickly and well they actually work.

Rose Oil

With several elements known to help with healing, this oil contains antimicrobials and anti-inflammatory properties. It also improves the texture and tone of your skin while improving skin conditions like psoriasis and dermatitis.

If you even just breathe this oil you're going to feel less stress and when you feel less stress you will have far fewer breakouts and far fewer wrinkles. The benefit is that you get to just stop and smell the roses. When you do you start feeling better right away. If your skin is dry or you are suffering from any skin conditions you can use this oil to help.

Example

Using these oils is going to help you best if you ingest them or use them topically. Some of the oils, like rose and myrrh, are going to be best when used topically because they help you to improve your skin from the outside while frankincense, for example, is great when ingested because it helps to improve the skin cells from the inside out.

You'll start to experience great benefits using them in these ways because you're going to help them reach the areas that they benefit a lot faster.

Word of Caution

Make sure you're diluting these oils properly, especially if you're ingesting them or applying them to your skin. It can be very dangerous to use these oils in too strong of a concentration so you want to make sure that you have them properly diluted as we talked about earlier.

Also, make sure that you're using pure oils as your additive because the synthetic ones could contain chemicals that are unhealthy for you or for your children if they happen to be around you. Make sure that you are really careful to keep them from getting into your eyes or nose while applying as well.

Exercise #7

For this exercise you want to use one of your new oils topically to improve your skin. Make sure to dilute it with a pure oil or moisturizer before applying it to your skin. You want to actually massage it in even if you're not actually using it for massage because this is going to help your skin absorb it.

Apply the oil mixture to your hand and then gently rub it into the skin in a circular motion. This is going to help you get as much of the oil as possible into the areas you're having trouble with. You'll also be able to smell the oil all day which will help with stress and other aspects at the same time.

Chapter 8: Using Essential Oils for Overcoming Addictions

What You'll Learn

Many people suffer from addictions and it's nothing to be ashamed about. If you're reading this chapter then it means you're trying to better yourself and you're trying to improve your addictions naturally.

You want to make yourself a better person by getting rid of those addictions and getting back to your life. Well there are a number of different essential oils that are able to help you with this very noble goal.

All you need to do is make sure you're using them the right way and you're going to reduce the cravings and side effects that go along with stopping use of an addictive substance.

Step by Step Description

Lavender Oil

There are many ways that lavender oil will help to improve your overall health and this is extremely important when attempting to overcome an addiction. Now for many of the things you suffer while you're coming off an addiction this oil can benefit.

It's great for helping with anxiety as well as withdrawal, two of the most dangerous aspects of your addiction; no matter what you happen to be addicted to. It can help to relieve some of the stress through this process and you will be able to relax and devote more of your time and energy to other things rather than the withdrawal symptoms.

Geranium Oil

This is oil that will have several benefits if you're trying to overcome an addiction. You'll have less trouble with sex or work addictions by using this particular oil, which can be dangerous or troubling addictions for many people.

Because work addictions can cost someone just as much as other addictions, resulting in a loss of the family, they are also important to be discussed in this section. Consider how much better your life would be if you weren't obsessed with one thing all the time? That's exactly what this oil will do no matter how it is used.

Basil Oil

Best for caffeine, drug and work addictions, and basil will also help you to feel more relaxed. It's great for a variety of different applications and can be used in a number of different ways. If you are looking for a way to energize your body you will also want to use this oil because it's perfect for refreshing and clarifying the mind and body altogether.
You'll feel a lot better all-around because this oil affects your entire perception about yourself and about anything around you at the same time.

Grapefruit Oil

A great way to take care of many different aspects of your addiction all at the same time, this oil actually works for cravings, withdrawal, caffeine addictions, drug addictions, food addictions and sugar addictions.

So when you use this one you're going to start feeling a lot better. If you have any of these addictions you're going to feel better faster and if you're just suffering from withdrawal or cravings you're going to get a bit of relief from those as well. Whether you inhale these oils or you ingest them you're going to get the benefits that we've mentioned and more.

Orange Oil

This oil works best for those with work addictions or anyone that is suffering from withdrawal. You'll be able to ease your condition this way and you're going to feel a lot better about your ability to quit your addiction.

What you need to do is inhale or ingest this oil and you'll be able to reduce the negative side effects of your withdrawal. Going without whatever you are addicted to is going to be difficult but you don't have to just give up. You can use these oils to help you reduce the cravings themselves and start getting back to your life.

Example

The best way to use essential oils if you are suffering from an addiction is through diffusing them. If you add the oil to a diffuser you'll start experiencing benefits from them almost right away. You start to breathe in the oils and this can help to calm your mind and relax the side effects that you are feeling.

You want to use these oils in this manner because it's going to cause a lot of change in a short time without you needing to wait for them to be absorbed by the body, your mind recognizes the benefits almost immediately.

Word of Caution

It's important to moderate your intake of oils. Even though you're not actually ingesting them you are going to get a lot of them into your system because your body starts to absorb them as you use the diffuser. Anything that is around your body will be absorbed through the skin, after all.

So make sure that you're using smaller amounts of these oils and that you're not continuing to diffuse them throughout your home for the entire day. This could result in health problems instead of fixing your health problems. If you have asthma you should also be careful about using oils in a diffuser as it could aggravate the condition.

Exercise #8

For this exercise, take out your favorite oil and just take a whiff of the scent.

How does it make you feel?

Do you feel energized?

Maybe you feel relaxed?

Does it evoke a memory in you?

Your sense of smell is actually strongly tied to your memory so it's likely that the smell will evoke memories of a vacation, a special meal or anything at all. Think about why you associate that smell with that memory and why it makes you feel the way that it does.

These aspects are going to greatly improve the way that you feel about different oils and how much they help you. Go through different oils and write down your memories or feelings based on the smell. You may actually have additional benefits for some oils because of these memories and feelings that are specific only to you.

Chapter 9: Using Essential Oils for Anti-Aging

What You'll Learn

No one likes to get older. In fact, as a society we spend millions of dollars attempting to look younger. What you may not even have realized is that essential oils are able to help you improve your skin and make you look younger.

You'll be able to get rid of a lot of wrinkles, reduce lines, reduce discoloration and more simply by using these oils in different ways. Often they are great when used topically but some don't even require that to achieve the benefits that you really want and need.

Step by Step Description

Sandalwood Oil

Looking to reduce aging? Well this is a great oil for it because you're going to get your skin more moisturized as well as reducing wrinkles. You'll be able to develop new skin cells more easily and will also improve your circulation.

When blood circulation improves it can dramatically improve the way that your skin looks and it can improve the elasticity as well as the look of those lines immensely as well. You're going to have smoother skin and you'll have less need for another moisturizing cream. Just apply a little sandalwood oil instead.

Myrrh Oil

Anti-fungal and anti-bacterial, myrrh will reduce your wrinkles, especially those located near your eyes. You will reduce levels of free radicals which can increase these wrinkles and you're going to get more skin cell repair at the same time.

You will even get benefits from the antioxidants that are in this oil and you're going to love the scent all at the same time. You can use this as a massage oil or you can apply it topically to the skin if you're looking for the best benefits from wrinkle prevention and removal.

Neroli Oil

This is a great oil to improve your skins elasticity. It helps to make your skin softer and more youthful which means that it's going to bounce back a lot better than it did before. As a result of this you're going to have a lot less wrinkles and you'll also experience less aging.

It's soothing and calming oil which also means that you're going to feel a lot more relaxed as you use it. So not only are you going to look better when you look in that mirror but you're actually going to feel a lot better and a lot calmer at the same time.

Clary Sage Oil

If you want to get rid of those wrinkles and lines then you want sage oil. It can be used with regular moisturizers to help tighten up your pores and improve your skin tone. It will even improve the texture of your skin which makes it look a lot smoother.

This contributes to a much younger look and will help you feel a lot better about yourself. No one wants to look old, so being able to get rid of all those wrinkles is definitely going to improve the way you feel about yourself. It's also going to help you feel more centered.

Geranium Oil

The final oil to use is one that you're probably already using but don't even realize it. It's actually been used in cosmetics for a long time and it helps to improve the blood circulation of your body.

It can improve the elasticity in the skin and will help you no matter what skin type you may have. If you're looking to get rid of sagging skin on the face this is the oil for you because it improves moisture content. It's best used as a massage oil to help improve these benefits.

Example

Using your oils to improve your aging process is great because you're going to look better and feel better about yourself. The best way to do this is to topically apply these oils. They're going to help you best when applied directly to wrinkles or dark spots.

You'll be surprised how much these oils actually improve the way that you look and you're definitely going to be surprised with how you get to look when you keep using them. Make sure to dilute them with other products as well so you are not getting them too strong as this could cause problems from skin irritation.

Word of Caution

If you have high blood pressure, history of convulsions or you're pregnant it's important consult your doctor before using a variety of different oils. They can interact negatively with your condition or with medications that you may be on to help the condition. If you know you have these conditions or even if you're not sure you will want to talk with a doctor and you'll be able to improve your health. You want to make sure that you don't mix anything that could be harmful.

Exercise #9

For this chapter take one of your oils and mix it with some water to create a cleaning solution. You can use this to wipe down your house or you can put a cotton ball soaked in the solution in your vacuum to impart some of the scent to your floors.

This is going to help you feel better about yourself because you get the scent at all times. It will literally be coming out of your floors.

That means your house is going to smell great and it's going to improve your wellbeing whether it's your stress levels, mind clarity or anything else.

Chapter 10: Using Essential Oils for Respiratory Systems

What You'll Learn

There are a large number of people that suffer from respiratory conditions. Different essential oils can be great for helping with these conditions because they actually help you to breathe a little better by clearing your airways.

Of course, you'll want to make sure that you're using these oils properly if you're going to do this because anything that affects your breathing will also have the ability to hurt your breathing.

Step by Step Description

Peppermint Oil

A scent and flavor that has long been used by those with breathing problems, peppermint oil works by cooling the respiratory system which helps it to dilate. This makes it much easier for you to breathe so you can continue on with your day.

If you're looking for additional health benefits you'll be happy to know that this oil is also antiseptic and anti-inflammatory, meaning that it will help you with any type of medical problem you might be experiencing. You'll start to feel better very quickly and you can do so by inhaling or ingesting this oil.

Lemon Oil

You'll start feeling a lot better because this oil actually improves your mental and emotional abilities. When you are struggling for breath this can be a great thing because it helps you to relax your body and to feel more in tune with the things that are happening around you.

You'll even be able to heal better, warm yourself and improve the air quality around you as well with the use of this oil. Of course, it smells pretty good too with the traditional citrusy aroma that we all associate with lemons whether smelling or cooking them.

Bay Laurel Oil

Antiseptic and antifungal, this oil will improve anything from asthma and bronchitis to viral infections. You'll feel better because you're able to breathe much easier and you'll also reduce fever and toxins in your body.

This means the oil will actually help you feel great in a variety of different ways, being a great all-around healer for your body. You will have less hair loss, muscle loss and spasms as well as a better appetite and less pain relief. All of this can be beneficial if you have a disorder or disease that is causing problems with your respiratory system.

Eucalyptus Oil

This oil actually improves respiratory problems very well by reducing inflammation in the nasal mucous membrane. This helps to reduce problems with colds as well as throat irritation. You'll even be able to reduce the viral infections in your body because this oil is perfect for combatting them.

To help improve your respiratory system even further it acts as a decongestant and an antibacterial. If you need older benefits it will improve your brain strength, skin, teeth, injuries and fever or muscle pain. If you have diabetes it's also an excellent oil for helping reduce the problems associated with this disorder.

Tea Tree Oil

Finally, this oil is intended to help with bronchitis, coughing and inflammation because it is an antibacterial, antifungal and antiviral. This is on top of its antimicrobial and stimulant nature. It can reduce septicity in wounds, improve the absorption of nutrients, reduce healing time on any type of injury and even kill insects when used properly.

You can use this oil for just about anything around you and you can even use it to improve the regular functions of your body. Just make sure you use it if you're feeling ill because it will definitely help you to feel better no matter what ails you.

Example

One of the best ways you can use oils when you have respiratory problems is to breathe them in. Because they work by clearing out your throat, your nose and airways you're actually helping to get rid of some of the blockage which can help you breathe better.

You also have the ability to ingest these oils in order to get the same types of benefits. For example, many people will use peppermint candies to help them with breathing problems. Natural oils will help these conditions even more.

Word of Caution

Talk with your doctor before you start using these oils. They can definitely improve your health and help you breathe better, but they can also cause you some health problems if not used properly.

Your doctor will be able to let you know if using these through diffusion is actually going to be best for you or if you should try another method. They can also help you understand what these oils are going to do for you when used in other ways.

Exercise #10

For this chapter, take your favorite essential oil and put it in your diffuser. Now take at least five to ten minutes to relax and just breathe it in. Place the diffuser close to you and slowly breathe in and out with your eyes closed.

Let the scent envelop you and let it take you wherever it will. This may sound a little strange but you'll start to feel something as a result of the oil and the scent. It will make you remember some place or something and you'll be able to truly relax your mind and body which will energize you for whatever else you need to do.

Chapter 11: Amazing Essential Oil Recipes

What You'll Learn

In this chapter we're going to talk about some great essential oil recipes. We'll explain what you need to do in order to use these oils properly and why you're going to want to use them through your life in order to help you feel better and be better in all aspects of your life. You don't need to spend a lot of your time and effort on it but the more you allow yourself to feel better with essential oils the better you're actually going to feel all around. So don't wait.

Step by Step How to Do It

Diffuser Recipe #1
4 drops Rose
4 drops Lavender
8 drops Mandarin
4 drops Vetiver

Improves anxiety and helps to calm the mind.

Diffuser Recipe #2
12 drops Lavender
8 drops Clary Sage

Helps reduce anxiety and clear the mind.

Body Lotion
8 ounces of unscented body lotion
20 drops Sandalwood
10 drops Patchouli
5 drops Carrot Seed

Mix together to improve dry skin and get a rich but smooth scent.

Antibiotic Cream
3 ounces Vegetable Oil (all natural)
1 ounce Beeswax (grated)
40 drops Lavender & Tea Tree Oils

4 ounce jar

Melt the beeswax carefully while also heating your oil. Put the warm oil into a bowl with the beeswax and stir then add other ingredients. Pour into jar while still warm and wait to cool before closing the container. You should wait for the oil to cool before using it.

Massage Oil #1
1 ounce all-natural oil
6 drops Clary Sage
2 Drops Lemon & Lavender Oils

Mix the oils together for a massage oil that will help to relieve stress and reduce your anxiety levels.

Massage Oil #2
1 ounce all-natural oil
2 drops Ginger
4 drops Peppermint
1 drop Black Pepper
5 drops Eucalyptus

Mix together for a muscle relaxant blend.

Carpet Cleaner
20 drops Lemon
40 drops Lavender
32 ounces Baking Soda

Mix together and apply to carpet just like you were applying body powder. Let it sit for a few moments before vacuuming.

Word of Caution

Remember that essential oils really can be somewhat dangerous if you don't use them properly. If you see something that says to dilute an oil then you definitely need to do it. Don't allow yourself to skip over this process because you could cause yourself or your family harm.

Diluting aromatherapy oils is how you're going to keep yourself from getting skin irritations through use. Also, make sure that you speak with your doctor about whether or not it is safe for you to use essential oils at all so you don't end up hurting yourself.

Exercise #11

For this final exercise it's time to create your routine. Look through the different chapters we've given you and look over the chapter at the end of the book where we talk about some of the essential oils and what they're used for.

Figure out which ones you like the best and create a list of your go-to oils for different things. Find one for when you're a little depressed and need a pick-me-up and one for when you need to relax. Maybe you'll find one for when you're not feeling well. This list is going to help you whenever you feel the need to improve yourself in any way.

Conclusion

There are a number of different ways that you can use essential oils and you'll want to consider several of them. No matter what conditions you may have or how you want to improve your abilities you will be able to do so with essential oils. Now that you know the best essential oils for specific situations you'll be able to use them even better.

What you want to do is make sure you're choosing the right essential oils for your condition. You can use many of them for different things, but keep in mind that you're also going to want to get the ones that are going to help what you're suffering from.

Whether you need something for memory improvement or you're looking for something that will help you look younger again, there's an essential oil for absolutely any need. If you need them for something we haven't discussed just look in the last chapter. You'll no doubt find something there.

The key to using essential oils is paying attention to your body. You'll know what you need and you'll be able to figure out how best to use it as well. Take a moment to speak with your doctor about any conditions you might have, just to make sure you're going to be safe using essential oils.

Next, make sure you're getting true essential oils and then make sure that you are using them. They can't help you if you aren't going to use them after all.

*Bonus *Chapter 12: More Tips & Techniques

Make sure you get real essential oils and not perfume oils. You won't get the same type of benefits from perfume oils which are only intended to provide an aroma.

Make sure you get oils in glass bottles only. The entire bottle should be glass with no rubber as this can ruin the oils.

Make sure your oils are entirely pure so you don't end up with synthetic chemicals which can harm you or your family.

Make sure you're researching different recipes that you can use for oils as they are going to be used in a variety of different methods. You can use them in many ways but want to make sure you get the recipe right.

Compare botanical names to ensure you are comparing exactly the same product from different suppliers if you're trying to choose the right one. Different botanical names could actually be entirely different oils.

Find out what type of 'farm' the oils are gathered from. You can usually find out the right country and then find out what type of oil gathering is used, which can affect the quality of the oil.

Purchase your oils from reputable persons who are going to get you high quality products. Don't buy from people at fairs or craft shows because you may not get what you're really looking for.

Make sure your oil is stored in dark glass bottles as this will keep the oils from diluting. The bottles should also be stored somewhere cool and dark.

Make sure you pay attention to any safety information that is included with your oils to keep from getting hurt.

You can order oils online and there are many reputable companies that you can do so with. Make sure that your company is good and gives only quality materials. This is going to help you save a little money.

For inhalation use only 1 or 2 drops of water on a tissue.

For a bath add only 8-10 drops into a full bath.

For a cleanser use 20 drops with 4 ounces of another product.

If you're using with a vacuum cleaner use 5-10 drops.

Add 10-20 drops to a washing machine per load

Some of the best oils to use with your essential oils are olive oil, jojoba oil, almond oil, grapeseed oil, coconut oil or avocado oil.

Extra Bonus Chapter 13: All the Essential Oils

There are a large number of different essential oils and understanding each one and how it can benefit you is definitely important so you can aid any problems you may have.

1. Allspice– With a warm, spicy-sweet scent, this is actually used as a more masculine scent. It actually helps with cheering, comforting and nurturing whoever uses it.

2. Angelica –Angelica is a good for digestive, expectorant, and stimulant. It can help you purify your blood, reduce gas, relax spasm, and improve perspiration rates.

3. Anise-Anise has been used a medicinal for centuries for reasons including anti-hysteric, expectorant, stimulant, and an anti-spasmodic. Anise could be useful to clear congestion, relax spasm, and treat arthritis pain.

4. Basil, Sweet-Basil is considered for use as an antibacterial and analgesic. It can promote healthy skin, blood circulation, and fix indigestion.

5. Bay-Oil from bay leaves can be used for many things including a sedative, antibiotic, and an analgesic. This can benefit you by reducing a fever, calm inflammation, and has been known to stop hair loss.

6. Benzoin- This oil can be used as an antidepressant, deodorant, relaxant, or anti-inflammatory device. It's useful to stop gas, helping cure infections, and as a depression fighter.

7. Bergamot-Bergamot has a variety of uses including an antibiotic, analgesic, and a disinfectant. Benefits of it include

using it to suppress pain, heal over scars, and reduce body odor.

8. Birch-Oil from birch has been used as a disinfectant, analgesic, and as an antiseptic. Use of birch can stop pain, reduce fever, and purify blood.

9. Bitter Almond-Almond oil can be used as an anesthetic, a diuretic, or as a sedative. Bitter Almond has benefits including being a desensitizing agent, can help you restore regularity, and as an anti-inflammatory.

10. Black Pepper-Oil from black pepper plants has been used as to help digestion, as an anti-arthritic, and an antibacterial agent. Some specific benefits include reducing gas, helping treat spasms, and fighting premature aging.

11. Buchu- This is used mainly as an antiseptic, anti-arthritic, and a diuretic. This can help reduce rheumatism and arthritis, increase digestive health, and can protect against the symptoms of being septic.

12. Cajuput-Oil of Cajuput has been used as a decongestant, expectorant, and as a stimulant. This can help you reduce pain, congestion, and fever.

13. Calamus-Using this can be good for your circulatory system, improve memory, and could be used as a tranquilizer. Calamus can help induce sleep, improve memory and brain function and increase circulation.

14. Camphor, White-Camphor oil could be used as a disinfectant, decongestant, and as an anesthetic. Properties like this could help you by being a local anesthetic, reduce congestion, and help decrease inflammation.

15. Caraway-Oil from Caraway has been known to be a diuretic, expectorant and as a stimulant. It's been used to increase hearth health, reduce gas, and fight infections.

16. Cardamom Seed-Oil of Cardamom seed has been used to reduce nausea, be a stimulant, and been used to combat the adverse effects of chemotherapy. Some other benefits include a wound protector, promote healthy digestion, and increase urination.

17. Carrot Seed-Carrot seed oil can be used as an antioxidant, a stimulant, and a disinfectant. This can be used for reducing gas, purifying the blood, and increase cell regeneration.

18. Cassia Bark-This can be used as an antidepressant, an anti-diarrheal, an astringent. It can help maintain regularity, slow the loss of hair and reduce hemorrhaging.

19. Catnip-Generally used for cats as the name suggest it also has uses for humans including as stimulant, an antispasmodic, and an astringent. That could mean benefits of reducing spasms, increase nervous system activity, and maintain stomach health.

20. Cedarwood, Red-Oil from cedarwood has been used as an antiseptic, expectorant and as a sedative. It has been used to fight off coughs and colds, regulate inflammation, and calm inflammation.

21. Chamomile-This oil is an antispasmodic, antiseptic, antibiotic, antiphlogistic and sedative. It can be used to cure spasms, protect wounds, eliminate gas, decrease visibility of scars, aid in digestion and kill bacteria. It also increases perspiration fights off infections and relieves inflammation.

22. Cinnamon-Cinnamon oil could be used as an antimicrobial, an anti-clotting and an antibacterial agent. Oil from cinnamon can be used to alleviate respiratory problems, heal wounds and pain, and can fix indigestion.

23. Citronella-Citronella is more than just a mosquito repellant as it can be used as an antibacterial, antiseptic, and a diuretic. You could benefit from use of it by its properties that can reduce spasm, stop inflammation, and regulate digestive health.

24. Clary Sage-Use of this is considered an antiseptic, sedative and an astringent. Things it can alleviate include righting depression, slow bacterial growth, and lower blood pressure.

25. Clove Bud-Oil from the clove has been used as an antimicrobial, antiviral, and an antiseptic. Use of the oil can reduce headaches and earaches, increase blood circulation, and improve the immune system.

26. Coriander Seed-Another oil that is derived from a spice or herb plant; coriander has been used as a stimulant, analgesic, and an antispasmodic. It can help reduce pain, reduce gas and regulate digestion.

27. Cumin-This oil has been used as a diuretic, antiseptic and a stimulant. Cumin can be used to reduce gas, regulate the digestive system and purify blood.

28. Cypress-Cypress oil is an antiseptic, diuretic and a sedative. It can help strengthen gums, calm spasm, and increase respiratory activity.

29. Davana-This oil is an antidepressant as well as an antiseptic, antiviral and disinfectant. It can be used for fighting depression, lifting your mood and protecting against wounds. It's also great for relieving menstrual cycles, relaxing the body and improving your mind.

30. Dill-Dill oil is an antispasmodic, digestive, disinfectant and sedative. It can be used for relieving spasms, promoting healthy digestion, soothing anxiety and increasing perspiration.

31. Elemi-Great for use as an antiseptic, analgesic and stimulant, Elemi also relieves pain, increases muscle tone and your overall health.

32. Eucalyptus-This oil is an anti-inflammatory, antispasmodic, decongestant, deodorant, antiseptic and antibacterial. It can be used to treat respiratory problems, wounds, muscle pain, dental care, skin care, fever and intestinal problems.

33. Fennel-Used an antiseptic, antispasmodic, diuretic, laxative, tonic and stimulant. It is used for protecting wounds, increasing appetite, purifying blood, increasing milk secretion, relieving constipation and relieving stomach problems.

34. Frankincense-This is used an antiseptic, disinfectant, diuretic, digestive, sedative and tonic. It is used for fighting infections, keeping cells healthy, promoting digestion, regulating menstrual cycles and curing colds.

35. Galbanum-This oil is an antispasmodic, decongestant, emollient, insecticide and antiparasitic. It's used to treat arthritis, removing scars, improving blood circulation, killing insects, improving wound healing and easing breathing.

36. Geranium-A quality astringent, diuretic, deodorant and tonic, geranium is used to tighten muscles, heal scars, improve cell growth and stop body odor.

37. Ginger-Ginger is an analgesic, antiseptic, antispasmodic, laxative and tonic. It relaxes spasms, stops vomiting, eliminates gas and improves brain function. It also helps to break fevers and improves color in the skin.

38. Grapefruit-This oil is a diuretic, disinfectant, stimulant, antidepressant and antiseptic. It's used to fight infections, reducing depression, protecting wounds and eliminating toxins.

39. Helicrysum-This oil is an antispasmodic, anticoagulant, antimicrobial, anti-inflammatory, antiseptic or diuretic. It's used to fight allergies, dissolve blood clots, reducing inflammation from fever, healing scars and protecting wounds.

40. Hyssop-This oil is an astringent, stimulant, digestive, diuretic, hypertensive, tonic and expectorant. It also tightens muscles and skin, eliminating gas, promoting digestion, increasing blood pressure, promoting sweating and reducing fever.

41. Jasmine-This oil is an antidepressant, antiseptic, aphrodisiac, antispasmodic, expectorant and sedative. It can be used for fighting depression, protecting wounds, regulating menstrual cycles, sedating inflammation and eases labor pains.

42. Juniper-This oil is an antiseptic, stimulant, astringent and diuretic. It will increase sweating, purifying blood, reducing gas, improving color in the skin and promoting wound healing.

43. Lavandin-Lavandin is an antidepressant, antiseptic, analgesic and expectorant. It fights depression, protects wounds from developing, reducing pain and healing scars.

44. Lavender-This oil is actually very calming and induces sleep. It's also an analgesic, disinfectant, anti-inflammatory,

antiseptic and antifungal. It is good for relieving nervous system disorders, pain relief and infection. It also cures fevers and stops hair lice.

45. Lemon-Lemon oil is an antiseptic, antiviral, astringent, bactericidal, disinfectant and restorative. It is great for stopping hair loss, inducing firm muscles and fighting infections.

46. Lemongrass-This oil is an analgesic, antidepressant, antimicrobial, antiseptic, astringent, bactericidal, deodorant, diuretic and sedative. It's used to fight depression, inhibit microbial growth, reduce hemorrhaging, kill bacteria, stop fungal infection and sooth inflammation.

47. Lime-Lime is used as an antiseptic, antiviral, astringent, disinfectant and restorative. It's used to protect against infection, boost appetite and kill bacteria as well as stopping hemorrhaging.

48. Mandarin-This oil is an antiseptic, antispasmodic, digestive, relaxant and sedative. It's used for purifying blood, increasing lymph circulation, improving liver health and soothing inflammation.

49. Manuka-This oil is an antidandruff, antibacterial, antifungal, anti-inflammatory, antihistaminic and deodorant. It is used to counter bites, cure fungal infections, sedate inflammation, reduce allergic symptoms and clear scars.

50. Marjoram-This oil is an analgesic, antispasmodic, anaphrodisiac, antiseptic, antiviral, digestive, diuretic and laxative. It's used to enhance libido, remove gas, cure constipation, kill fungus, cure headaches.

51. Melissa-This oil is an antidepressant, sedative, antispasmodic, antibacterial and tonic. It's used to reduce depression, inhibit bacteria, remove gas, remove toxins and reduce fever.

52. Mugwort-This mugwort is used as a digestive, diuretic, stimulant and uterine. It's used for digestion, removing toxins, treating nervous disorders, maintaining uterine health and killing intestinal worms.

53. Mullein-This oil is an analgesic, anti-inflammatory, antiseptic, disinfectant and diuretic. It protects wounds, eases inflammation, fights infections and removes toxins from your body.

54. Mustard-This oil is a stimulant, irritant, antibacterial, antifungal, insect repellant and tonic. It is used to increase appetite, keep insects away, boost hair growth, reduce hair loss, boost health and stimulate circulation.

55. Myrrh-This oil is an antimicrobial, astringent, expectorant, antifungal, stimulant, antiseptic, immune booster and anti-inflammatory. It's used to alleviate colds, stop fungal growth, promote sweating, boost protection against diseases and improve circulation.

56. Myrtle-This is an antiseptic, astringent, deodorant and sedative. It's used for wound healing, tight gums, reducing body odor, fighting colds and soothing inflammation.

57. Neroli-This oil is an antidepressant, aphrodisiac, antiseptic, disinfectant, antispasmodic, deodorant, digestive and sedative. It's used to enhance libido, protecting wounds, kill bacteria, reducing spasms, fighting infections and eliminating body odor.

58. Niaouli-This oil is an analgesic, antiseptic, decongestant, insecticide and stimulant. It is used for rheumatism, arthritis, protecting wounds, boosting health, decreasing congestion and reducing fever.

59. Nutmeg-This oil is an analgesic, antiemetic, antioxidant, antiseptic, antispasmodic, antiparasitic and aphrodisiac. It's

used to relieve pain, stop premature aging, protect wounds, enhance libido and improve heart health.

60. Oakmoss-This oil is an antiseptic, expectorant and restorative. It's used to improve wounds, restore health and expel phlegm.

61. Orange-This oil is an anti-inflammatory, antidepressant, antispasmodic, antiseptic and aphrodisiac. This oil is used to soothe inflammation, fight depression, enhance libido and tone your general health and immune system.

62. Oregano-This oil is an antiviral, antibacterial, antifungal, antiparasitic, antioxidant, anti-inflammatory and digestive. It's used to improve inflammation, promote digestion and cure allergies.

63. Palma Rosa-This oil is an antiseptic, antiviral, digestive and hydration balm. It's used to inhibit viral growth facilitate digestion and reduce fever.

64. Parsley-This oil is an antimicrobial, antiarthritic, digestive, diuretic, depurative and laxative. It is used to treat rheumatism, stop hair loss, improve blood circulation, remove toxins, purify blood and clear the bowels.

65. Patchouli-This oil is an antidepressant, antiphlogistic, antiseptic, astringent, deodorant, diuretic and fungicide. It can be used to fight depression, improve mood, soothe fever, protect wounds, stop hemorrhaging, remove toxins and kill insects.

66. Pennyroyal-This oil is an antimicrobial, antibacterial, antirheumatic, antiseptic, astringent, decongestant and digestive. It is used to stop bacterial growth, treat arthritis, prevent hair loss, clear congestion and purify blood as well as easing breathing.

67. Peppermint-This oil is an analgesic, anesthetic, antiseptic, antispasmodic, astringent, decongestant, hepatic, stimulant and sudorific. It is used to treat pain, reduce milk flow, relieve spasms, improve memory health, ease breathing, reduce fever and improve the liver and nerves.

68. Petitgrain-This oil is an antiseptic, antispasmodic, antidepressant and deodorant. It is used to relax spasms, fight off depression, improve mood and get rid of body odor.

69. Pimento-This oil is an anaesthetic, analgesic, antioxidant, antiseptic and stimulant. It is used to promote numbness, reduce pain, reduce premature aging, color the skin and relax the entire body and mind.

70. Pine-Uses as an antibacterial, analgesic, diuretic and antiseptic, this oil is used for skin care and cosmetics. It also relieves pain, stress and mental fatigue.

71. Ravensara-An excellent analgesic, anti-allergenic, antibacterial, antimicrobial, antidepressant, antifungal, antiseptic, antispasmodic and antiviral, this oil is used for pain relief, improving allergies, fighting off depression, increasing libido and improving the mood.

72. Rose-This oil is an antidepressant, antiseptic, antispasmodic, antiviral, aphrodisiac, astringent, laxative and stomachic. It is used to fight depression, improve the mood, protect wounds, cure sexual disorders, inhibit bacterial growth, purify the blood and stop hemorrhaging.

73. Rosemary-A disinfectant, antiseptic, anti-inflammatory and antibacterial, this oil is used to improve hair growth, skin care, mouth care, depression and rheumatism. It is also used to reduce respiratory problems, indigestion and flatulence.

74. Rosewood-This oil is an analgesic, antidepressant, antiseptic, aphrodisiac, antibacterial, deodorant and insecticide. It is

used to reduce pain, fight depression, kill bacteria, improve the brain and cure headaches.

75. Rue-This oil is an antiarthritic, antirheumatic, antibacterial, antifungal and insecticidal. It is used to neutralize poisons, inhibit bacterial, kill insects, sooth nervous afflictions and promote digestion.

76. Sage-This oil is an antifungal, antimicrobial, antibacterial, antiseptic, antioxidant, anti-inflammatory, digestive and disinfectant. It is used to protect wounds, heal damages, soothe inflammation, clear spasms and promote digestion.

77. Sandalwood-This oil is an antiseptic, anti-inflammatory, antispasmodic, astringent, diuretic and disinfectant. It is used to tighten gums, stop hair loss, fight infection, smooth out the skin and remove infections.

78. Spearmint-This oil is an antiseptic, antispasmodic, insecticide and restorative. It is used to protect against wounds, clear spasms, relieve gas and kill insects.

79. Spikenard-This oil is an antibacterial, antifungal, anti-inflammatory, deodorant and laxative. It is used to relieve inflammation, eliminate body odor and clear the bowels. It is used to relieve nervous afflictions.

80. Tagetes-This oil is an antibiotic, antimicrobial, antiparasitic, antiseptic, antispasmodic, disinfectant and insecticide. It is used to purify the blood, reduce inflammation and reduce nervous disorders.

81. Tangerine-This oil is an antiseptic, antispasmodic, sedative and tonic. It is used to reduce inflammation, purify blood, regenerate cells and reduce nervous disorders.

82. Tansy-This oil is an antibacterial, antifungal, anti-inflammatory, antiviral, insecticide and sedative. It is used

for relieving inflammation, repelling insects, fixing nervous afflictions and reducing fever.

83. Tarragon-This oil is an antirheumatic, digestive, deodorant and stimulant. It is used to treat arthritis, improve blood circulation, improve digestion, kill intestinal worms and inhibit bacterial infections.

84. Tea Tree-This oil is an antibacterial, antimicrobial, antiviral, fungicide, insecticide and antiseptic. It is used to protect wounds, kill insects, heal scars and cure colds. It is even used to stimulate systemic functions and discharges.

85. Thuja-This oil is an antirheumatic, astringent, diuretic, expectorant, insect repellent and tonic. It used to stop hair loss, reduce hemorrhage, remove toxins, repel insects, tone up the entire body.

86. Thyme-This oil is an antispasmodic, antiseptic, diuretic, expectorant and stimulant. It is used to protect wounds, kill bacteria, cure chest infections, relieve gas, heal scars and regulate the menstrual cycle.

87. Tuberose-This oil is an aphrodisiac, deodorant, relaxant and sedative. It is used to enhance libido, get rid of body odor, soothe inflammation and reduce any type of nervous disorders.

88. Vanilla-This oil is an antioxidant, aphrodisiac, antidepressant, sedative and tranquilizer. It is used to enhance libido, fight off depression, lift mood and relieve anxiety. It is also used to promote sleep and relieve stress.

89. Vetiver-This oil is an anti-inflammatory, antiseptic, aphrodisiac and sedative. It is used to relieve inflammation, increase libido, heal scars and fix nervous disorders.

90. Wintergreen-This oil is an analgesic, antiarthritic antispasmodic, antiseptic and aromatic. It's used to relax the

body, reduce hair loss, reduce hemorrhaging, and relieve toxins.

91. Wormwood-This oil is an deodorant, digestive, insecticide and tonic. It is used to kill worms, get rid of body odor, get rid of digestion, relieve fever and kill insects.

92. Yarrow-This oil is an anti-inflammatory, antirheumatic, antiseptic, astringent, digestive and tonic. It is used to stop hemorrhaging, relieve gas, heal scars, relieve coughs and lower blood pressure.

93. Ylang Ylang Extra-This oil is an antidepressant, antiseptic and aphrodisiac. It is used to increase libido and cure sexual disorders as well as helping with nervous disorders and reducing blood pressure.

www.ingramcontent.com/pod-product-compliance
Lightning Source LLC
Chambersburg PA
CBHW070323290526
45791CB00003B/1233